THIS JOURNAL BELONGS TO:

_____

PUBLISHED BY: ADIL DAISY

DATE      HOT   COLD   MILD

 START TIME   🏁 **END TIME**

TOTAL DURATION   **TOTAL DISTANCE**

ELEVATION GAIN/LOSS

TRAIL TYPE (CIRCLE ONE): ○ **OUT & BACK**   ○ **LOOP**   ○ **ONE WAY / SHUTTLE**

📍 THE HIKE ☆☆☆☆☆

CITY/STATE

TRAIL(S)

START LATITUDE/LONGITUDE

TERRAIN

CEL PHONE RECEPTION/CARRIER

○ **FIRST VISIT**   ○ **RETURN VISIT**

PERSONAL RATING: ○ **EASY**   ○ **INTERMEDIATE**   ○ **DIFICULT**

 COMPANION(S)

FACILITIES / WATER AVAIABILITY

TRAIL & WEATHER CONDITIONS

OBSERVANCES (WILDLIFE, NATURE, VIEWS, ETC)

NOTES FOR NEXT TIME (SHUTTLES, ENTRANCE FEES, PARKING, ROUTES, PETS, ETC.)

HIKING NOTES

_____

_____

_____

_____

_____

_____

_____

_____

_____

_____

_____

TRAIL DRAWING / FAVORITE PHOTO

DATE   HOT COLD MILD

 START TIME   **END TIME**

TOTAL DURATION   **TOTAL DISTANCE**

ELEVATION GAIN/LOSS

TRAIL TYPE (CIRCLE ONE):   ◯ OUT & BACK   ◯ LOOP   ◯ ONE WAY / SHUTTLE

📍 THE HIKE   ☆ ☆ ☆ ☆ ☆

CITY/STATE

TRAIL(S)

START LATITUDE/LONGITUDE

TERRAIN

CEL PHONE RECEPTION/CARRIER

◯ **FIRST VISIT**   ◯ **RETURN VISIT**

PERSONAL RATING: ◯ EASY   ◯ INTERMEDIATE   ◯ DIFICULT

 COMPANION(S)

FACILITIES / WATER AVAIABILITY

TRAIL & WEATHER CONDITIONS

OBSERVANCES (WILDLIFE, NATURE, VIEWS, ETC)

NOTES FOR NEXT TIME (SHUTTLES, ENTRANCE FEES, PARKING, ROUTES, PETS, ETC.)

HIKING NOTES

_____

_____

_____

_____

_____

_____

_____

_____

_____

_____

_____

TRAIL DRAWING / FAVORITE PHOTO

DATE 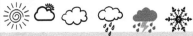 **HOT** **COLD** **MILD**

START TIME **END TIME**

TOTAL DURATION _____ **TOTAL DISTANCE** _____

ELEVATION GAIN/LOSS _____

TRAIL TYPE (CIRCLE ONE): ◯ **OUT & BACK** ◯ **LOOP** ◯ **ONE WAY / SHUTTLE**

THE HIKE ★ ★ ★ ★

CITY/STATE _____

TRAIL(S) _____

START LATITUDE/LONGITUDE _____

TERRAIN _____

CEL PHONE RECEPTION/CARRIER _____

◯ **FIRST VISIT** ◯ **RETURN VISIT**

PERSONAL RATING: ◯ **EASY** ◯ **INTERMEDIATE** ◯ **DIFICULT**

 COMPANION(S) _____

_____

FACILITIES / WATER AVAIABILITY _____

_____

TRAIL & WEATHER CONDITIONS _____

_____

OBSERVANCES (WILDLIFE, NATURE, VIEWS, ETC) _____

_____

NOTES FOR NEXT TIME (SHUTTLES, ENTRANCE FEES, PARKING, ROUTES, PETS, ETC.) _____

_____

HIKING NOTES

_____

_____

_____

_____

_____

_____

_____

_____

_____

_____

_____

TRAIL DRAWING / FAVORITE PHOTO

DATE 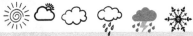 HOT COLD MILD

 START TIME **END TIME**

TOTAL DURATION **TOTAL DISTANCE**

ELEVATION GAIN/LOSS

TRAIL TYPE (CIRCLE ONE): ○ **OUT & BACK** ○ **LOOP** ○ **ONE WAY / SHUTTLE**

 # THE HIKE ★★★★★

CITY/STATE

TRAIL(S)

START LATITUDE/LONGITUDE

TERRAIN

CEL PHONE RECEPTION/CARRIER

○ **FIRST VISIT** ○ **RETURN VISIT**

PERSONAL RATING: ○ **EASY** ○ **INTERMEDIATE** ○ **DIFICULT**

 COMPANION(S)

FACILITIES / WATER AVAIABILITY

TRAIL & WEATHER CONDITIONS

OBSERVANCES (WILDLIFE, NATURE, VIEWS, ETC)

NOTES FOR NEXT TIME (SHUTTLES, ENTRANCE FEES, PARKING, ROUTES, PETS, ETC.)

HIKING NOTES

_____
_____
_____
_____
_____
_____
_____
_____
_____
_____
_____

TRAIL DRAWING / FAVORITE PHOTO

DATE   HOT COLD MILD

START TIME **END TIME**

TOTAL DURATION   **TOTAL DISTANCE**

ELEVATION GAIN/LOSS

TRAIL TYPE (CIRCLE ONE):   OUT & BACK   LOOP   ONE WAY / SHUTTLE

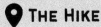 ## THE HIKE ⭐⭐⭐⭐⭐

CITY/STATE

TRAIL(S)

START LATITUDE/LONGITUDE

TERRAIN

CEL PHONE RECEPTION/CARRIER

FIRST VISIT   RETURN VISIT

PERSONAL RATING: EASY   INTERMEDIATE   DIFICULT

 COMPANION(S)

FACILITIES / WATER AVAIABILITY

TRAIL & WEATHER CONDITIONS

OBSERVANCES (WILDLIFE, NATURE, VIEWS, ETC)

NOTES FOR NEXT TIME (SHUTTLES, ENTRANCE FEES, PARKING, ROUTES, PETS, ETC.)

HIKING NOTES

_____

_____

_____

_____

_____

_____

_____

_____

_____

_____

_____

_____

_____

TRAIL DRAWING / FAVORITE PHOTO

DATE  HOT   COLD   MILD

 START TIME 🏁 **END TIME**

TOTAL DURATION **TOTAL DISTANCE**

ELEVATION GAIN/LOSS

TRAIL TYPE (CIRCLE ONE): ○ **OUT & BACK** ○ **LOOP** ○ **ONE WAY / SHUTTLE**

📍 THE HIKE ⭐⭐⭐⭐⭐

CITY/STATE

TRAIL(S)

START LATITUDE/LONGITUDE

TERRAIN

CEL PHONE RECEPTION/CARRIER

○ **FIRST VISIT** ○ **RETURN VISIT**

PERSONAL RATING: ○ **EASY** ○ **INTERMEDIATE** ○ **DIFICULT**

 COMPANION(S)

FACILITIES / WATER AVAIABILITY

TRAIL & WEATHER CONDITIONS

OBSERVANCES (WILDLIFE, NATURE, VIEWS, ETC)

NOTES FOR NEXT TIME (SHUTTLES, ENTRANCE FEES, PARKING, ROUTES, PETS, ETC.)

HIKING NOTES

_____

_____

_____

_____

_____

_____

_____

_____

_____

_____

_____

_____

TRAIL DRAWING / FAVORITE PHOTO

DATE 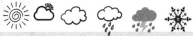 HOT COLD MILD

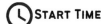 **START TIME** **END TIME**

TOTAL DURATION   **TOTAL DISTANCE**

ELEVATION GAIN/LOSS

TRAIL TYPE (CIRCLE ONE):   ◯ **OUT & BACK**   ◯ **LOOP**   ◯ **ONE WAY / SHUTTLE**

THE HIKE   ☆ ☆ ☆ ☆ ☆

CITY/STATE

TRAIL(S)

START LATITUDE/LONGITUDE

TERRAIN

CEL PHONE RECEPTION/CARRIER

◯ **FIRST VISIT**   ◯ **RETURN VISIT**

PERSONAL RATING: ◯ **EASY**   ◯ **INTERMEDIATE**   ◯ **DIFICULT**

 COMPANION(S)

FACILITIES / WATER AVAIABILITY

TRAIL & WEATHER CONDITIONS

OBSERVANCES (WILDLIFE, NATURE, VIEWS, ETC)

NOTES FOR NEXT TIME (SHUTTLES, ENTRANCE FEES, PARKING, ROUTES, PETS, ETC.)

HIKING NOTES

_____
_____
_____
_____
_____
_____
_____
_____
_____
_____
_____
_____

TRAIL DRAWING / FAVORITE PHOTO

DATE _____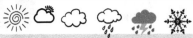

🕐 **START TIME** _____ 🏁 **END TIME** _____

TOTAL DURATION _____ **TOTAL DISTANCE** _____

ELEVATION GAIN/LOSS _____

TRAIL TYPE (CIRCLE ONE): ◯ **OUT & BACK** ◯ **LOOP** ◯ **ONE WAY / SHUTTLE**

📍 THE HIKE ⭐ ⭐ ⭐ ⭐ ⭐

CITY/STATE _____

TRAIL(S) _____

START LATITUDE/LONGITUDE _____

TERRAIN _____

CEL PHONE RECEPTION/CARRIER _____

◯ **FIRST VISIT** ◯ **RETURN VISIT**

PERSONAL RATING: ◯ **EASY** ◯ **INTERMEDIATE** ◯ **DIFICULT**

 COMPANION(S) _____

_____

FACILITIES / WATER AVAIABILITY _____

_____

TRAIL & WEATHER CONDITIONS _____

_____

OBSERVANCES (WILDLIFE, NATURE, VIEWS, ETC) _____

_____

NOTES FOR NEXT TIME (SHUTTLES, ENTRANCE FEES, PARKING, ROUTES, PETS, ETC.) _____

_____

HIKING NOTES

_____

_____

_____

_____

_____

_____

_____

_____

_____

_____

_____

TRAIL DRAWING / FAVORITE PHOTO

DATE _____ 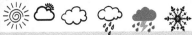 **HOT** **COLD** **MILD**

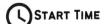 **START TIME** _____ 🏁 **END TIME** _____

TOTAL DURATION _____ **TOTAL DISTANCE** _____

ELEVATION GAIN/LOSS _____

TRAIL TYPE (CIRCLE ONE): ○ **OUT & BACK**   ○ **LOOP**   ○ **ONE WAY / SHUTTLE**

📍 THE HIKE ⭐⭐⭐⭐⭐

CITY/STATE _____

TRAIL(S) _____

START LATITUDE/LONGITUDE _____

TERRAIN _____

CEL PHONE RECEPTION/CARRIER _____

○ **FIRST VISIT**   ○ **RETURN VISIT**

PERSONAL RATING: ○ **EASY**   ○ **INTERMEDIATE**   ○ **DIFICULT**

 COMPANION(S) _____

_____

FACILITIES / WATER AVAIABILITY _____

_____

TRAIL & WEATHER CONDITIONS _____

_____

OBSERVANCES (WILDLIFE, NATURE, VIEWS, ETC) _____

_____

NOTES FOR NEXT TIME (SHUTTLES, ENTRANCE FEES, PARKING, ROUTES, PETS, ETC.) _____

_____

HIKING NOTES

_____
_____
_____
_____
_____
_____
_____
_____
_____
_____
_____
_____

TRAIL DRAWING / FAVORITE PHOTO

DATE 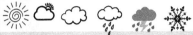 **HOT** **COLD** **MILD**

 START TIME   **END TIME**

TOTAL DURATION   **TOTAL DISTANCE**

ELEVATION GAIN/LOSS

TRAIL TYPE (CIRCLE ONE):   **OUT & BACK**   **LOOP**   **ONE WAY / SHUTTLE**

THE HIKE ⭐⭐⭐⭐⭐

CITY/STATE

TRAIL(S)

START LATITUDE/LONGITUDE

TERRAIN

CEL PHONE RECEPTION/CARRIER

    FIRST VISIT   **RETURN VISIT**

PERSONAL RATING: **EASY**   **INTERMEDIATE**   **DIFICULT**

 COMPANION(S)

FACILITIES / WATER AVAIABILITY

TRAIL & WEATHER CONDITIONS

OBSERVANCES (WILDLIFE, NATURE, VIEWS, ETC)

NOTES FOR NEXT TIME (SHUTTLES, ENTRANCE FEES, PARKING, ROUTES, PETS, ETC.)

HIKING NOTES

_____

_____

_____

_____

_____

_____

_____

_____

_____

_____

_____

TRAIL DRAWING / FAVORITE PHOTO

Date   **Hot** **Cold** **Mild**

Start Time **End Time**

Total Duration   **Total Distance**

Elevation Gain/Loss

Trail Type (Circle One):   ◯ **Out & Back**   ◯ **Loop**   ◯ **One Way / Shuttle**

📍 The Hike   ★ ★ ★ ★ ★

City/State

Trail(s)

Start Latitude/Longitude

Terrain

Cel Phone Reception/Carrier

◯ **First Visit**   ◯ **Return Visit**

Personal Rating: ◯ **Easy**   ◯ **Intermediate**   ◯ **Dificult**

 Companion(s)

_____

Facilities / Water Avaiability

_____

Trail & Weather Conditions

_____

Observances (Wildlife, Nature, Views, Etc)

_____

Notes For Next Time (Shuttles, Entrance fees, Parking, Routes, Pets, Etc.)

_____

HIKING NOTES

_____

_____

_____

_____

_____

_____

_____

_____

_____

_____

_____

_____

TRAIL DRAWING / FAVORITE PHOTO

Date 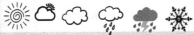 **Hot** **Cold** **Mild**

Start Time **End Time**

Total Duration _____ **Total Distance** _____

Elevation Gain/Loss _____

Trail Type (Circle One): ◯ **Out & Back** ◯ **Loop** ◯ **One Way / Shuttle**

The Hike ☆ ☆ ☆ ☆ ☆

City/State _____

Trail(s) _____

Start Latitude/Longitude _____

Terrain _____

Cel Phone Reception/Carrier _____

◯ **First Visit** ◯ **Return Visit**

Personal Rating: ◯ **Easy** ◯ **Intermediate** ◯ **Dificult**

 Companion(s)

_____

Facilities / Water Avaiability

_____

Trail & Weather Conditions

_____

Observances (Wildlife, Nature, Views, Etc)

_____

Notes For Next Time (Shuttles, Entrance fees, Parking, Routes, Pets, Etc.)

_____

HIKING NOTES

_____
_____
_____
_____
_____
_____
_____
_____
_____
_____
_____
_____
_____
_____

TRAIL DRAWING / FAVORITE PHOTO

DATE 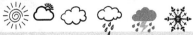 HOT COLD MILD

START TIME **END TIME**

TOTAL DURATION   **TOTAL DISTANCE**

ELEVATION GAIN/LOSS

TRAIL TYPE (CIRCLE ONE):   OUT & BACK   LOOP   ONE WAY / SHUTTLE

 THE HIKE   ⭐ ⭐ ⭐ ⭐ ⭐

CITY/STATE

TRAIL(S)

START LATITUDE/LONGITUDE

TERRAIN

CEL PHONE RECEPTION/CARRIER

     FIRST VISIT   **RETURN VISIT**

PERSONAL RATING: EASY   INTERMEDIATE   DIFICULT

 COMPANION(S)

FACILITIES / WATER AVAIABILITY

TRAIL & WEATHER CONDITIONS

OBSERVANCES (WILDLIFE, NATURE, VIEWS, ETC)

NOTES FOR NEXT TIME (SHUTTLES, ENTRANCE FEES, PARKING, ROUTES, PETS, ETC.)

HIKING NOTES

_____
_____
_____
_____
_____
_____
_____
_____
_____
_____
_____
_____

TRAIL DRAWING / FAVORITE PHOTO

Date 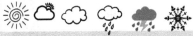 HOT COLD MILD

Start Time **End Time**

Total Duration   **Total Distance**

Elevation Gain/Loss

Trail Type (Circle One):   ○ **Out & Back**   ○ **Loop**   ○ **One Way / Shuttle**

 ## The Hike   ☆ ☆ ☆ ☆ ☆

City/State

Trail(s)

Start Latitude/Longitude

Terrain

Cel Phone Reception/Carrier

○ **First Visit**   ○ **Return Visit**

Personal Rating: ○ **Easy**   ○ **Intermediate**   ○ **Dificult**

 Companion(s)

Facilities / Water Avaiability

Trail & Weather Conditions

Observances (Wildlife, Nature, Views, Etc)

Notes For Next Time (Shuttles, Entrance fees, Parking, Routes, Pets, Etc.)

HIKING NOTES

_____
_____
_____
_____
_____
_____
_____
_____
_____
_____
_____
_____

TRAIL DRAWING / FAVORITE PHOTO

DATE 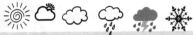 HOT COLD MILD

START TIME **END TIME**

TOTAL DURATION   **TOTAL DISTANCE**

ELEVATION GAIN/LOSS

TRAIL TYPE (CIRCLE ONE): ◯ **OUT & BACK** ◯ **LOOP** ◯ **ONE WAY / SHUTTLE**

THE HIKE ☆ ☆ ☆ ☆ ☆

CITY/STATE

TRAIL(S)

START LATITUDE/LONGITUDE

TERRAIN

CEL PHONE RECEPTION/CARRIER

◯ **FIRST VISIT**   ◯ **RETURN VISIT**

PERSONAL RATING: ◯ **EASY** ◯ **INTERMEDIATE** ◯ **DIFICULT**

 COMPANION(S)

FACILITIES / WATER AVAIABILITY

TRAIL & WEATHER CONDITIONS

OBSERVANCES (WILDLIFE, NATURE, VIEWS, ETC)

NOTES FOR NEXT TIME (SHUTTLES, ENTRANCE FEES, PARKING, ROUTES, PETS, ETC.)

HIKING NOTES

_____

_____

_____

_____

_____

_____

_____

_____

_____

_____

_____

_____

_____

TRAIL DRAWING / FAVORITE PHOTO

DATE

START TIME **END TIME**

TOTAL DURATION _____ **TOTAL DISTANCE** _____

ELEVATION GAIN/LOSS _____

TRAIL TYPE (CIRCLE ONE): ◯ **OUT & BACK** ◯ **LOOP** ◯ **ONE WAY / SHUTTLE**

 THE HIKE ★ ★ ★ ★ ★

CITY/STATE _____

TRAIL(S) _____

START LATITUDE/LONGITUDE _____

TERRAIN _____

CEL PHONE RECEPTION/CARRIER _____

◯ **FIRST VISIT** ◯ **RETURN VISIT**

PERSONAL RATING: ◯ **EASY** ◯ **INTERMEDIATE** ◯ **DIFICULT**

 COMPANION(S)

_____

FACILITIES / WATER AVAIABILITY

_____

TRAIL & WEATHER CONDITIONS

_____

OBSERVANCES (WILDLIFE, NATURE, VIEWS, ETC)

_____

NOTES FOR NEXT TIME (SHUTTLES, ENTRANCE FEES, PARKING, ROUTES, PETS, ETC.)

_____

HIKING NOTES

_____
_____
_____
_____
_____
_____
_____
_____
_____
_____
_____
_____
_____
_____

TRAIL DRAWING / FAVORITE PHOTO

DATE 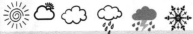   HOT COLD MILD

🕐 **START TIME** 🏁 **END TIME**

TOTAL DURATION _____ **TOTAL DISTANCE** _____

ELEVATION GAIN/LOSS _____

TRAIL TYPE (CIRCLE ONE): ⚪ **OUT & BACK** ⚪ **LOOP** ⚪ **ONE WAY / SHUTTLE**

📍 THE HIKE ⭐⭐⭐⭐⭐

CITY/STATE _____

TRAIL(S) _____

START LATITUDE/LONGITUDE _____

TERRAIN _____

CEL PHONE RECEPTION/CARRIER _____

⚪ **FIRST VISIT** ⚪ **RETURN VISIT**

PERSONAL RATING: ⚪ **EASY** ⚪ **INTERMEDIATE** ⚪ **DIFICULT**

 COMPANION(S) _____
_____

FACILITIES / WATER AVAIABILITY _____
_____

TRAIL & WEATHER CONDITIONS _____
_____

OBSERVANCES (WILDLIFE, NATURE, VIEWS, ETC) _____
_____

NOTES FOR NEXT TIME (SHUTTLES, ENTRANCE FEES, PARKING, ROUTES, PETS, ETC.) _____
_____

HIKING NOTES

_____
_____
_____
_____
_____
_____
_____
_____
_____
_____
_____
_____
_____

TRAIL DRAWING / FAVORITE PHOTO

DATE  HOT COLD MILD

START TIME **END TIME**

TOTAL DURATION   **TOTAL DISTANCE**

ELEVATION GAIN/LOSS

TRAIL TYPE (CIRCLE ONE):   ○ **OUT & BACK**   ○ **LOOP**   ○ **ONE WAY / SHUTTLE**

 THE HIKE ⭐⭐⭐⭐⭐

CITY/STATE

TRAIL(S)

START LATITUDE/LONGITUDE

TERRAIN

CEL PHONE RECEPTION/CARRIER

○ **FIRST VISIT**   ○ **RETURN VISIT**

PERSONAL RATING: ○ **EASY**   ○ **INTERMEDIATE**   ○ **DIFICULT**

 COMPANION(S)

FACILITIES / WATER AVAIABILITY

TRAIL & WEATHER CONDITIONS

OBSERVANCES (WILDLIFE, NATURE, VIEWS, ETC)

NOTES FOR NEXT TIME (SHUTTLES, ENTRANCE FEES, PARKING, ROUTES, PETS, ETC.)

HIKING NOTES

(blank lined notes section)

TRAIL DRAWING / FAVORITE PHOTO

DATE _____  HOT COLD MILD

 START TIME _____ **END TIME** _____

TOTAL DURATION _____ **TOTAL DISTANCE** _____

ELEVATION GAIN/LOSS _____

TRAIL TYPE (CIRCLE ONE): ⭕ OUT & BACK ⭕ LOOP ⭕ ONE WAY / SHUTTLE

📍 THE HIKE ⭐⭐⭐⭐⭐

CITY/STATE _____

TRAIL(S) _____

START LATITUDE/LONGITUDE _____

TERRAIN _____

CEL PHONE RECEPTION/CARRIER _____

⭕ FIRST VISIT ⭕ RETURN VISIT

PERSONAL RATING: ⭕ EASY ⭕ INTERMEDIATE ⭕ DIFICULT

 COMPANION(S)
_____
_____

FACILITIES / WATER AVAIABILITY
_____
_____

TRAIL & WEATHER CONDITIONS
_____
_____

OBSERVANCES (WILDLIFE, NATURE, VIEWS, ETC)
_____
_____

NOTES FOR NEXT TIME (SHUTTLES, ENTRANCE FEES, PARKING, ROUTES, PETS, ETC.)
_____
_____

HIKING NOTES

_____
_____
_____
_____
_____
_____
_____
_____
_____
_____
_____
_____

TRAIL DRAWING / FAVORITE PHOTO

DATE   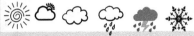 HOT COLD MILD

START TIME   **END TIME**

TOTAL DURATION   **TOTAL DISTANCE**

ELEVATION GAIN/LOSS

TRAIL TYPE (CIRCLE ONE):   ◯ **OUT & BACK**   ◯ **LOOP**   ◯ **ONE WAY / SHUTTLE**

 **THE HIKE**   ★ ★ ★ ★ ★

CITY/STATE

TRAIL(S)

START LATITUDE/LONGITUDE

TERRAIN

CEL PHONE RECEPTION/CARRIER

◯ **FIRST VISIT**   ◯ **RETURN VISIT**

PERSONAL RATING: ◯ **EASY**   ◯ **INTERMEDIATE**   ◯ **DIFICULT**

 COMPANION(S)

FACILITIES / WATER AVAIABILITY

TRAIL & WEATHER CONDITIONS

OBSERVANCES (WILDLIFE, NATURE, VIEWS, ETC)

NOTES FOR NEXT TIME (SHUTTLES, ENTRANCE FEES, PARKING, ROUTES, PETS, ETC.)

HIKING NOTES

TRAIL DRAWING / FAVORITE PHOTO

DATE 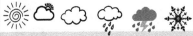 HOT COLD MILD

 START TIME   🏁 **END TIME**

TOTAL DURATION   **TOTAL DISTANCE**

ELEVATION GAIN/LOSS

TRAIL TYPE (CIRCLE ONE): ⬭ **OUT & BACK** ⬭ **LOOP** ⬭ **ONE WAY / SHUTTLE**

📍 **THE HIKE** ⭐ ⭐ ⭐ ⭐ ⭐

CITY/STATE

TRAIL(S)

START LATITUDE/LONGITUDE

TERRAIN

CEL PHONE RECEPTION/CARRIER

⬭ **FIRST VISIT**   ⬭ **RETURN VISIT**

PERSONAL RATING: ⬭ **EASY** ⬭ **INTERMEDIATE** ⬭ **DIFICULT**

 COMPANION(S)

FACILITIES / WATER AVAIABILITY

TRAIL & WEATHER CONDITIONS

OBSERVANCES (WILDLIFE, NATURE, VIEWS, ETC)

NOTES FOR NEXT TIME (SHUTTLES, ENTRANCE FEES, PARKING, ROUTES, PETS, ETC.)

HIKING NOTES

_____
_____
_____
_____
_____
_____
_____
_____
_____
_____
_____
_____
_____

TRAIL DRAWING / FAVORITE PHOTO

DATE   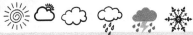 **HOT** **COLD** **MILD**

START TIME **END TIME**

TOTAL DURATION **TOTAL DISTANCE**

ELEVATION GAIN/LOSS

TRAIL TYPE (CIRCLE ONE): ◯ **OUT & BACK** ◯ **LOOP** ◯ **ONE WAY / SHUTTLE**

THE HIKE ☆ ☆ ☆ ☆ ☆

CITY/STATE

TRAIL(S)

START LATITUDE/LONGITUDE

TERRAIN

CEL PHONE RECEPTION/CARRIER

◯ **FIRST VISIT** ◯ **RETURN VISIT**

PERSONAL RATING: ◯ **EASY** ◯ **INTERMEDIATE** ◯ **DIFICULT**

 COMPANION(S)

FACILITIES / WATER AVAIABILITY

TRAIL & WEATHER CONDITIONS

OBSERVANCES (WILDLIFE, NATURE, VIEWS, ETC)

NOTES FOR NEXT TIME (SHUTTLES, ENTRANCE FEES, PARKING, ROUTES, PETS, ETC.)

HIKING NOTES

TRAIL DRAWING / FAVORITE PHOTO

DATE 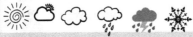 HOT COLD MILD

 START TIME   **END TIME**

TOTAL DURATION   **TOTAL DISTANCE**

ELEVATION GAIN/LOSS

TRAIL TYPE (CIRCLE ONE):   ○ **OUT & BACK**   ○ **LOOP**   ○ **ONE WAY / SHUTTLE**

 THE HIKE   ★ ★ ★ ★ ★

CITY/STATE

TRAIL(S)

START LATITUDE/LONGITUDE

TERRAIN

CEL PHONE RECEPTION/CARRIER

○ **FIRST VISIT**   ○ **RETURN VISIT**

PERSONAL RATING: ○ **EASY**   ○ **INTERMEDIATE**   ○ **DIFICULT**

 COMPANION(S)

FACILITIES / WATER AVAIABILITY

TRAIL & WEATHER CONDITIONS

OBSERVANCES (WILDLIFE, NATURE, VIEWS, ETC)

NOTES FOR NEXT TIME (SHUTTLES, ENTRANCE FEES, PARKING, ROUTES, PETS, ETC.)

HIKING NOTES

_____

_____

_____

_____

_____

_____

_____

_____

_____

_____

_____

TRAIL DRAWING / FAVORITE PHOTO

Date  HOT COLD MILD

⏱ **Start Time**   🏁 **End Time**

Total Duration   **Total Distance**

Elevation Gain/Loss

Trail Type (Circle One): ◯ **Out & Back** ◯ **Loop** ◯ **One Way / Shuttle**

📍 **The Hike** ⭐⭐⭐⭐⭐

City/State

Trail(s)

Start Latitude/Longitude

Terrain

Cel Phone Reception/Carrier

◯ **First Visit**   ◯ **Return Visit**

Personal Rating: ◯ **Easy** ◯ **Intermediate** ◯ **Dificult**

 Companion(s)

Facilities / Water Avaiability

Trail & Weather Conditions

Observances (Wildlife, Nature, Views, Etc)

Notes For Next Time (Shuttles, Entrance fees, Parking, Routes, Pets, Etc.)

HIKING NOTES

_____

_____

_____

_____

_____

_____

_____

_____

_____

_____

_____

_____

TRAIL DRAWING / FAVORITE PHOTO

DATE 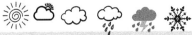 **HOT** **COLD** **MILD**

START TIME **END TIME**

TOTAL DURATION _____ **TOTAL DISTANCE** _____

ELEVATION GAIN/LOSS _____

TRAIL TYPE (CIRCLE ONE): ◯ **OUT & BACK** ◯ **LOOP** ◯ **ONE WAY / SHUTTLE**

 THE HIKE ☆ ☆ ☆ ☆ ☆

CITY/STATE _____

TRAIL(S) _____

START LATITUDE/LONGITUDE _____

TERRAIN _____

CEL PHONE RECEPTION/CARRIER _____

◯ **FIRST VISIT** ◯ **RETURN VISIT**

PERSONAL RATING: ◯ **EASY** ◯ **INTERMEDIATE** ◯ **DIFICULT**

 COMPANION(S) _____

_____

FACILITIES / WATER AVAIABILITY _____

_____

TRAIL & WEATHER CONDITIONS _____

_____

OBSERVANCES (WILDLIFE, NATURE, VIEWS, ETC) _____

_____

NOTES FOR NEXT TIME (SHUTTLES, ENTRANCE FEES, PARKING, ROUTES, PETS, ETC.) _____

_____

HIKING NOTES

_____
_____
_____
_____
_____
_____
_____
_____
_____
_____
_____
_____
_____

TRAIL DRAWING / FAVORITE PHOTO

DATE  HOT COLD MILD

START TIME **END TIME**

TOTAL DURATION   **TOTAL DISTANCE**

ELEVATION GAIN/LOSS

TRAIL TYPE (CIRCLE ONE):   OUT & BACK   LOOP   ONE WAY / SHUTTLE

 THE HIKE   ★ ★ ★ ★ ★

CITY/STATE

TRAIL(S)

START LATITUDE/LONGITUDE

TERRAIN

CEL PHONE RECEPTION/CARRIER

FIRST VISIT   RETURN VISIT

PERSONAL RATING: EASY   INTERMEDIATE   DIFICULT

 COMPANION(S)

FACILITIES / WATER AVAIABILITY

TRAIL & WEATHER CONDITIONS

OBSERVANCES (WILDLIFE, NATURE, VIEWS, ETC)

NOTES FOR NEXT TIME (SHUTTLES, ENTRANCE FEES, PARKING, ROUTES, PETS, ETC.)

HIKING NOTES

_____
_____
_____
_____
_____
_____
_____
_____
_____
_____
_____
_____

TRAIL DRAWING / FAVORITE PHOTO

DATE  **HOT** **COLD** **MILD**

 START TIME   **END TIME**

TOTAL DURATION   **TOTAL DISTANCE**

ELEVATION GAIN/LOSS

TRAIL TYPE (CIRCLE ONE):   ○ **OUT & BACK**   ○ **LOOP**   ○ **ONE WAY / SHUTTLE**

THE HIKE ⭐⭐⭐⭐⭐

CITY/STATE

TRAIL(S)

START LATITUDE/LONGITUDE

TERRAIN

CEL PHONE RECEPTION/CARRIER

    ○ **FIRST VISIT**   ○ **RETURN VISIT**

PERSONAL RATING: ○ **EASY**   ○ **INTERMEDIATE**   ○ **DIFICULT**

 COMPANION(S)

FACILITIES / WATER AVAIABILITY

TRAIL & WEATHER CONDITIONS

OBSERVANCES (WILDLIFE, NATURE, VIEWS, ETC)

NOTES FOR NEXT TIME (SHUTTLES, ENTRANCE FEES, PARKING, ROUTES, PETS, ETC.)

HIKING NOTES

_____
_____
_____
_____
_____
_____
_____
_____
_____
_____
_____
_____
_____

TRAIL DRAWING / FAVORITE PHOTO

Date 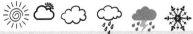 HOT COLD MILD

START TIME   **END TIME**

TOTAL DURATION   **TOTAL DISTANCE**

ELEVATION GAIN/LOSS

TRAIL TYPE (CIRCLE ONE):   OUT & BACK   LOOP   ONE WAY / SHUTTLE

 THE HIKE   ☆ ☆ ☆ ☆ ☆

CITY/STATE

TRAIL(S)

START LATITUDE/LONGITUDE

TERRAIN

CEL PHONE RECEPTION/CARRIER

FIRST VISIT   RETURN VISIT

PERSONAL RATING: EASY   INTERMEDIATE   DIFICULT

 COMPANION(S)

FACILITIES / WATER AVAIABILITY

TRAIL & WEATHER CONDITIONS

OBSERVANCES (WILDLIFE, NATURE, VIEWS, ETC)

NOTES FOR NEXT TIME (SHUTTLES, ENTRANCE FEES, PARKING, ROUTES, PETS, ETC.)

HIKING NOTES

_____

_____

_____

_____

_____

_____

_____

_____

_____

_____

_____

_____

_____

TRAIL DRAWING / FAVORITE PHOTO

Date   **HOT** **COLD** **MILD**

 Start Time **End Time**

Total Duration **Total Distance**

Elevation Gain/Loss

Trail Type (Circle One): ⭕ **Out & Back** ⭕ **Loop** ⭕ **One Way / Shuttle**

 The Hike ⭐ ⭐ ⭐ ⭐ ⭐

City/State

Trail(s)

Start Latitude/Longitude

Terrain

Cel Phone Reception/Carrier

⭕ **First Visit** ⭕ **Return Visit**

Personal Rating: ⭕ **Easy** ⭕ **Intermediate** ⭕ **Dificult**

 Companion(s)

Facilities / Water Avaiability

Trail & Weather Conditions

Observances (Wildlife, Nature, Views, Etc)

Notes For Next Time (Shuttles, Entrance fees, Parking, Routes, Pets, Etc.)

HIKING NOTES

TRAIL DRAWING / FAVORITE PHOTO

DATE _____ 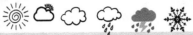 **HOT** **COLD** **MILD**

START TIME _____   **END TIME** _____

TOTAL DURATION _____   **TOTAL DISTANCE** _____

ELEVATION GAIN/LOSS _____

TRAIL TYPE (CIRCLE ONE):   ◯ **OUT & BACK**   ◯ **LOOP**   ◯ **ONE WAY / SHUTTLE**

 # THE HIKE   ★ ★ ★ ★ ★

CITY/STATE _____

TRAIL(S) _____

START LATITUDE/LONGITUDE _____

TERRAIN _____

CEL PHONE RECEPTION/CARRIER _____

◯ **FIRST VISIT**   ◯ **RETURN VISIT**

PERSONAL RATING: ◯ **EASY**   ◯ **INTERMEDIATE**   ◯ **DIFICULT**

 COMPANION(S) _____

_____

FACILITIES / WATER AVAIABILITY _____

_____

TRAIL & WEATHER CONDITIONS _____

_____

OBSERVANCES (WILDLIFE, NATURE, VIEWS, ETC) _____

_____

NOTES FOR NEXT TIME (SHUTTLES, ENTRANCE FEES, PARKING, ROUTES, PETS, ETC.) _____

_____

HIKING NOTES

_____

_____

_____

_____

_____

_____

_____

_____

_____

_____

_____

_____

_____

TRAIL DRAWING / FAVORITE PHOTO

DATE 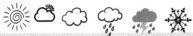 **HOT** **COLD** **MILD**

START TIME **END TIME**

TOTAL DURATION _____ **TOTAL DISTANCE** _____

ELEVATION GAIN/LOSS _____

TRAIL TYPE (CIRCLE ONE): ◯ **OUT & BACK** ◯ **LOOP** ◯ **ONE WAY / SHUTTLE**

THE HIKE ☆☆☆☆☆

CITY/STATE _____

TRAIL(S) _____

START LATITUDE/LONGITUDE _____

TERRAIN _____

CEL PHONE RECEPTION/CARRIER _____

◯ **FIRST VISIT** ◯ **RETURN VISIT**

PERSONAL RATING: ◯ **EASY** ◯ **INTERMEDIATE** ◯ **DIFICULT**

 COMPANION(S) _____

_____

FACILITIES / WATER AVAIABILITY _____

_____

TRAIL & WEATHER CONDITIONS _____

_____

OBSERVANCES (WILDLIFE, NATURE, VIEWS, ETC) _____

_____

NOTES FOR NEXT TIME (SHUTTLES, ENTRANCE FEES, PARKING, ROUTES, PETS, ETC.) _____

_____

HIKING NOTES

_____

_____

_____

_____

_____

_____

_____

_____

_____

_____

_____

_____

TRAIL DRAWING / FAVORITE PHOTO

DATE   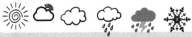   **HOT** **COLD** **MILD**

START TIME **END TIME**

TOTAL DURATION **TOTAL DISTANCE**

ELEVATION GAIN/LOSS

TRAIL TYPE (CIRCLE ONE): ◯ **OUT & BACK** ◯ **LOOP** ◯ **ONE WAY / SHUTTLE**

THE HIKE ★ ★ ★ ★ ★

CITY/STATE

TRAIL(S)

START LATITUDE/LONGITUDE

TERRAIN

CEL PHONE RECEPTION/CARRIER

◯ **FIRST VISIT** ◯ **RETURN VISIT**

PERSONAL RATING: ◯ **EASY** ◯ **INTERMEDIATE** ◯ **DIFICULT**

 COMPANION(S)

FACILITIES / WATER AVAIABILITY

TRAIL & WEATHER CONDITIONS

OBSERVANCES (WILDLIFE, NATURE, VIEWS, ETC)

NOTES FOR NEXT TIME (SHUTTLES, ENTRANCE FEES, PARKING, ROUTES, PETS, ETC.)

HIKING NOTES

_____
_____
_____
_____
_____
_____
_____
_____
_____
_____
_____
_____
_____

TRAIL DRAWING / FAVORITE PHOTO

DATE 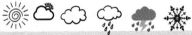 HOT COLD MILD

⏰ **START TIME** **END TIME**

TOTAL DURATION   **TOTAL DISTANCE**

ELEVATION GAIN/LOSS

TRAIL TYPE (CIRCLE ONE):   ⚪ **OUT & BACK**   ⚪ **LOOP**   ⚪ **ONE WAY / SHUTTLE**

📍 THE HIKE   ⭐⭐⭐⭐⭐

CITY/STATE

TRAIL(S)

START LATITUDE/LONGITUDE

TERRAIN

CEL PHONE RECEPTION/CARRIER

⚪ **FIRST VISIT**   ⚪ **RETURN VISIT**

PERSONAL RATING: ⚪ **EASY**   ⚪ **INTERMEDIATE**   ⚪ **DIFICULT**

 COMPANION(S)

FACILITIES / WATER AVAIABILITY

TRAIL & WEATHER CONDITIONS

OBSERVANCES (WILDLIFE, NATURE, VIEWS, ETC)

NOTES FOR NEXT TIME (SHUTTLES, ENTRANCE FEES, PARKING, ROUTES, PETS, ETC.)

HIKING NOTES

_____
_____
_____
_____
_____
_____
_____
_____
_____
_____
_____
_____
_____
_____

TRAIL DRAWING / FAVORITE PHOTO

DATE

START TIME **END TIME**

TOTAL DURATION _____ **TOTAL DISTANCE** _____

ELEVATION GAIN/LOSS _____

TRAIL TYPE (CIRCLE ONE): ◯ **OUT & BACK** ◯ **LOOP** ◯ **ONE WAY / SHUTTLE**

THE HIKE ☆☆☆☆☆

CITY/STATE _____

TRAIL(S) _____

START LATITUDE/LONGITUDE _____

TERRAIN _____

CEL PHONE RECEPTION/CARRIER _____

◯ **FIRST VISIT** ◯ **RETURN VISIT**

PERSONAL RATING: ◯ **EASY** ◯ **INTERMEDIATE** ◯ **DIFICULT**

 COMPANION(S) _____

_____

FACILITIES / WATER AVAIABILITY _____

_____

TRAIL & WEATHER CONDITIONS _____

_____

OBSERVANCES (WILDLIFE, NATURE, VIEWS, ETC) _____

_____

NOTES FOR NEXT TIME (SHUTTLES, ENTRANCE FEES, PARKING, ROUTES, PETS, ETC.)

_____

_____

HIKING NOTES

_____

_____

_____

_____

_____

_____

_____

_____

_____

_____

_____

_____

_____

TRAIL DRAWING / FAVORITE PHOTO

DATE  HOT COLD MILD

🕐 **START TIME**   🏁 **END TIME**

TOTAL DURATION   **TOTAL DISTANCE**

ELEVATION GAIN/LOSS

TRAIL TYPE (CIRCLE ONE): ⚪ **OUT & BACK** ⚪ **LOOP** ⚪ **ONE WAY / SHUTTLE**

📍 **THE HIKE**   ⭐⭐⭐⭐⭐

CITY/STATE

TRAIL(S)

START LATITUDE/LONGITUDE

TERRAIN

CEL PHONE RECEPTION/CARRIER

⚪ **FIRST VISIT**   ⚪ **RETURN VISIT**

PERSONAL RATING: ⚪ **EASY** ⚪ **INTERMEDIATE** ⚪ **DIFICULT**

 COMPANION(S)

FACILITIES / WATER AVAIABILITY

TRAIL & WEATHER CONDITIONS

OBSERVANCES (WILDLIFE, NATURE, VIEWS, ETC)

NOTES FOR NEXT TIME (SHUTTLES, ENTRANCE FEES, PARKING, ROUTES, PETS, ETC.)

HIKING NOTES

_____
_____
_____
_____
_____
_____
_____
_____
_____
_____
_____
_____

TRAIL DRAWING / FAVORITE PHOTO

DATE 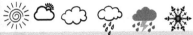 **HOT** **COLD** **MILD**

🕐 **START TIME** 🏁 **END TIME**

TOTAL DURATION **TOTAL DISTANCE**

ELEVATION GAIN/LOSS

TRAIL TYPE (CIRCLE ONE): ◯ **OUT & BACK** ◯ **LOOP** ◯ **ONE WAY / SHUTTLE**

📍 **THE HIKE** ⭐⭐⭐⭐⭐

CITY/STATE

TRAIL(S)

START LATITUDE/LONGITUDE

TERRAIN

CEL PHONE RECEPTION/CARRIER

◯ **FIRST VISIT** ◯ **RETURN VISIT**

PERSONAL RATING: ◯ **EASY** ◯ **INTERMEDIATE** ◯ **DIFICULT**

 COMPANION(S)

FACILITIES / WATER AVAIABILITY

TRAIL & WEATHER CONDITIONS

OBSERVANCES (WILDLIFE, NATURE, VIEWS, ETC)

NOTES FOR NEXT TIME (SHUTTLES, ENTRANCE FEES, PARKING, ROUTES, PETS, ETC.)

HIKING NOTES

TRAIL DRAWING / FAVORITE PHOTO

DATE |  **HOT** **COLD** **MILD**

 START TIME | **END TIME**

TOTAL DURATION | **TOTAL DISTANCE**

ELEVATION GAIN/LOSS

TRAIL TYPE (CIRCLE ONE): ○ **OUT & BACK** ○ **LOOP** ○ **ONE WAY / SHUTTLE**

 THE HIKE ☆☆☆☆☆

CITY/STATE

TRAIL(S)

START LATITUDE/LONGITUDE

TERRAIN

CEL PHONE RECEPTION/CARRIER

○ **FIRST VISIT** ○ **RETURN VISIT**

PERSONAL RATING: ○ **EASY** ○ **INTERMEDIATE** ○ **DIFICULT**

 COMPANION(S)

FACILITIES / WATER AVAIABILITY

TRAIL & WEATHER CONDITIONS

OBSERVANCES (WILDLIFE, NATURE, VIEWS, ETC)

NOTES FOR NEXT TIME (SHUTTLES, ENTRANCE FEES, PARKING, ROUTES, PETS, ETC.)

_____
_____
_____
_____
_____
_____
_____
_____
_____
_____
_____
_____

TRAIL DRAWING / FAVORITE PHOTO

DATE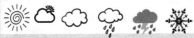

HOT   COLD   MILD

START TIME **END TIME**

TOTAL DURATION | **TOTAL DISTANCE**

ELEVATION GAIN/LOSS

TRAIL TYPE (CIRCLE ONE):   OUT & BACK   LOOP   ONE WAY / SHUTTLE

 THE HIKE   ★ ★ ★ ★ ★

CITY/STATE

TRAIL(S)

START LATITUDE/LONGITUDE

TERRAIN

CEL PHONE RECEPTION/CARRIER

   FIRST VISIT   RETURN VISIT

PERSONAL RATING: EASY   INTERMEDIATE   DIFICULT

 COMPANION(S)

FACILITIES / WATER AVAIABILITY

TRAIL & WEATHER CONDITIONS

OBSERVANCES (WILDLIFE, NATURE, VIEWS, ETC)

NOTES FOR NEXT TIME (SHUTTLES, ENTRANCE FEES, PARKING, ROUTES, PETS, ETC.)

TRAIL DRAWING / FAVORITE PHOTO

DATE 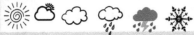 **HOT** **COLD** **MILD**

START TIME **END TIME**

TOTAL DURATION _____ **TOTAL DISTANCE** _____

ELEVATION GAIN/LOSS _____

TRAIL TYPE (CIRCLE ONE): ◯ **OUT & BACK** ◯ **LOOP** ◯ **ONE WAY / SHUTTLE**

◉ THE HIKE ★ ★ ★ ★ ★

CITY/STATE _____

TRAIL(S) _____

START LATITUDE/LONGITUDE _____

TERRAIN _____

CEL PHONE RECEPTION/CARRIER _____

◯ **FIRST VISIT** ◯ **RETURN VISIT**

PERSONAL RATING: ◯ **EASY** ◯ **INTERMEDIATE** ◯ **DIFICULT**

 COMPANION(S)

_____

_____

FACILITIES / WATER AVAIABILITY

_____

_____

TRAIL & WEATHER CONDITIONS

_____

_____

OBSERVANCES (WILDLIFE, NATURE, VIEWS, ETC)

_____

_____

NOTES FOR NEXT TIME (SHUTTLES, ENTRANCE FEES, PARKING, ROUTES, PETS, ETC.)

_____

_____

HIKING NOTES

_____
_____
_____
_____
_____
_____
_____
_____
_____
_____
_____
_____
_____
_____

TRAIL DRAWING / FAVORITE PHOTO

DATE _____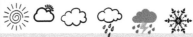

 START TIME _____ 🏁 **END TIME** _____

TOTAL DURATION _____ **TOTAL DISTANCE** _____

ELEVATION GAIN/LOSS _____

TRAIL TYPE (CIRCLE ONE): ○ **OUT & BACK** ○ **LOOP** ○ **ONE WAY / SHUTTLE**

📍 THE HIKE ⭐ ⭐ ⭐ ⭐ ⭐

CITY/STATE _____

TRAIL(S) _____

START LATITUDE/LONGITUDE _____

TERRAIN _____

CEL PHONE RECEPTION/CARRIER _____

○ **FIRST VISIT** ○ **RETURN VISIT**

PERSONAL RATING: ○ **EASY** ○ **INTERMEDIATE** ○ **DIFICULT**

 COMPANION(S)
_____
_____

FACILITIES / WATER AVAIABILITY
_____
_____

TRAIL & WEATHER CONDITIONS
_____
_____

OBSERVANCES (WILDLIFE, NATURE, VIEWS, ETC)
_____
_____

NOTES FOR NEXT TIME (SHUTTLES, ENTRANCE FEES, PARKING, ROUTES, PETS, ETC.)
_____
_____

HIKING NOTES

TRAIL DRAWING / FAVORITE PHOTO

DATE  **HOT** **COLD** **MILD**

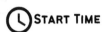 **START TIME**   **END TIME**

TOTAL DURATION   **TOTAL DISTANCE**

ELEVATION GAIN/LOSS

TRAIL TYPE (CIRCLE ONE):   OUT & BACK   LOOP   ONE WAY / SHUTTLE

 THE HIKE ⭐ ⭐ ⭐ ⭐ ⭐

CITY/STATE

TRAIL(S)

START LATITUDE/LONGITUDE

TERRAIN

CEL PHONE RECEPTION/CARRIER

    FIRST VISIT   RETURN VISIT

PERSONAL RATING: EASY   INTERMEDIATE   DIFICULT

 COMPANION(S)

FACILITIES / WATER AVAIABILITY

TRAIL & WEATHER CONDITIONS

OBSERVANCES (WILDLIFE, NATURE, VIEWS, ETC)

NOTES FOR NEXT TIME (SHUTTLES, ENTRANCE FEES, PARKING, ROUTES, PETS, ETC.)

HIKING NOTES

_____
_____
_____
_____
_____
_____
_____
_____
_____
_____
_____
_____

TRAIL DRAWING / FAVORITE PHOTO

DATE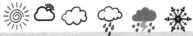

START TIME **END TIME**

TOTAL DURATION **TOTAL DISTANCE**

ELEVATION GAIN/LOSS

TRAIL TYPE (CIRCLE ONE): OUT & BACK LOOP ONE WAY / SHUTTLE

 THE HIKE ⭐⭐⭐⭐⭐

CITY/STATE

TRAIL(S)

START LATITUDE/LONGITUDE

TERRAIN

CEL PHONE RECEPTION/CARRIER

FIRST VISIT RETURN VISIT

PERSONAL RATING: EASY INTERMEDIATE DIFICULT

 COMPANION(S)

FACILITIES / WATER AVAIABILITY

TRAIL & WEATHER CONDITIONS

OBSERVANCES (WILDLIFE, NATURE, VIEWS, ETC)

NOTES FOR NEXT TIME (SHUTTLES, ENTRANCE FEES, PARKING, ROUTES, PETS, ETC.)

HIKING NOTES

_____
_____
_____
_____
_____
_____
_____
_____
_____
_____
_____

TRAIL DRAWING / FAVORITE PHOTO

DATE | 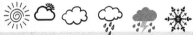 **HOT** **COLD** **MILD**

🕐 **START TIME** | 🏁 **END TIME**

TOTAL DURATION | **TOTAL DISTANCE**

ELEVATION GAIN/LOSS

TRAIL TYPE (CIRCLE ONE): ◯ **OUT & BACK** ◯ **LOOP** ◯ **ONE WAY / SHUTTLE**

📍 THE HIKE ⭐⭐⭐⭐⭐

CITY/STATE

TRAIL(S)

START LATITUDE/LONGITUDE

TERRAIN

CEL PHONE RECEPTION/CARRIER

◯ **FIRST VISIT** ◯ **RETURN VISIT**

PERSONAL RATING: ◯ **EASY** ◯ **INTERMEDIATE** ◯ **DIFICULT**

 COMPANION(S)

FACILITIES / WATER AVAIABILITY

TRAIL & WEATHER CONDITIONS

OBSERVANCES (WILDLIFE, NATURE, VIEWS, ETC)

NOTES FOR NEXT TIME (SHUTTLES, ENTRANCE FEES, PARKING, ROUTES, PETS, ETC.)

HIKING NOTES

_____
_____
_____
_____
_____
_____
_____
_____
_____
_____
_____
_____
_____

TRAIL DRAWING / FAVORITE PHOTO

DATE 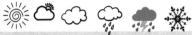 **HOT** **COLD** **MILD**

 START TIME **END TIME**

TOTAL DURATION **TOTAL DISTANCE**

ELEVATION GAIN/LOSS

TRAIL TYPE (CIRCLE ONE): ◯ **OUT & BACK** ◯ **LOOP** ◯ **ONE WAY / SHUTTLE**

 THE HIKE ☆ ☆ ☆ ☆ ☆

CITY/STATE

TRAIL(S)

START LATITUDE/LONGITUDE

TERRAIN

CEL PHONE RECEPTION/CARRIER

◯ **FIRST VISIT** ◯ **RETURN VISIT**

PERSONAL RATING: ◯ **EASY** ◯ **INTERMEDIATE** ◯ **DIFICULT**

 COMPANION(S)

FACILITIES / WATER AVAIABILITY

TRAIL & WEATHER CONDITIONS

OBSERVANCES (WILDLIFE, NATURE, VIEWS, ETC)

NOTES FOR NEXT TIME (SHUTTLES, ENTRANCE FEES, PARKING, ROUTES, PETS, ETC.)

HIKING NOTES

TRAIL DRAWING / FAVORITE PHOTO

DATE 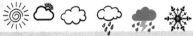 **HOT** **COLD** **MILD**

START TIME **END TIME**

TOTAL DURATION   **TOTAL DISTANCE**

ELEVATION GAIN/LOSS

TRAIL TYPE (CIRCLE ONE): ◯ **OUT & BACK**   ◯ **LOOP**   ◯ **ONE WAY / SHUTTLE**

 THE HIKE   ☆ ☆ ☆ ☆ ☆

CITY/STATE

TRAIL(S)

START LATITUDE/LONGITUDE

TERRAIN

CEL PHONE RECEPTION/CARRIER

◯ **FIRST VISIT**   ◯ **RETURN VISIT**

PERSONAL RATING: ◯ **EASY**   ◯ **INTERMEDIATE**   ◯ **DIFICULT**

 COMPANION(S)

FACILITIES / WATER AVAIABILITY

TRAIL & WEATHER CONDITIONS

OBSERVANCES (WILDLIFE, NATURE, VIEWS, ETC)

NOTES FOR NEXT TIME (SHUTTLES, ENTRANCE FEES, PARKING, ROUTES, PETS, ETC.)

HIKING NOTES

TRAIL DRAWING / FAVORITE PHOTO

DATE | 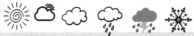 **HOT** **COLD** **MILD**

 START TIME   **END TIME**

TOTAL DURATION   **TOTAL DISTANCE**

ELEVATION GAIN/LOSS

TRAIL TYPE (CIRCLE ONE):   OUT & BACK   LOOP   ONE WAY / SHUTTLE

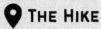 **THE HIKE**   ★ ★ ★ ★ ★

CITY/STATE

TRAIL(S)

START LATITUDE/LONGITUDE

TERRAIN

CEL PHONE RECEPTION/CARRIER

          FIRST VISIT   **RETURN VISIT**

PERSONAL RATING: EASY   INTERMEDIATE   DIFICULT

 COMPANION(S)

FACILITIES / WATER AVAIABILITY

TRAIL & WEATHER CONDITIONS

OBSERVANCES (WILDLIFE, NATURE, VIEWS, ETC)

NOTES FOR NEXT TIME (SHUTTLES, ENTRANCE FEES, PARKING, ROUTES, PETS, ETC.)

HIKING NOTES

_____

_____

_____

_____

_____

_____

_____

_____

_____

_____

_____

_____

_____

TRAIL DRAWING / FAVORITE PHOTO

DATE 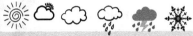 **HOT** **COLD** **MILD**

 START TIME   **END TIME**

TOTAL DURATION   **TOTAL DISTANCE**

ELEVATION GAIN/LOSS

TRAIL TYPE (CIRCLE ONE):   ○ **OUT & BACK**   ○ **LOOP**   ○ **ONE WAY / SHUTTLE**

THE HIKE   ★ ★ ★ ★ ★

CITY/STATE

TRAIL(S)

START LATITUDE/LONGITUDE

TERRAIN

CEL PHONE RECEPTION/CARRIER

○ **FIRST VISIT**   ○ **RETURN VISIT**

PERSONAL RATING: ○ **EASY**   ○ **INTERMEDIATE**   ○ **DIFICULT**

 COMPANION(S)

FACILITIES / WATER AVAIABILITY

TRAIL & WEATHER CONDITIONS

OBSERVANCES (WILDLIFE, NATURE, VIEWS, ETC)

NOTES FOR NEXT TIME (SHUTTLES, ENTRANCE FEES, PARKING, ROUTES, PETS, ETC.)

HIKING NOTES

_____
_____
_____
_____
_____
_____
_____
_____
_____
_____
_____
_____
_____
_____

TRAIL DRAWING / FAVORITE PHOTO

DATE 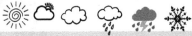 HOT COLD MILD

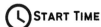 **START TIME**   🏁 **END TIME**

TOTAL DURATION   **TOTAL DISTANCE**

ELEVATION GAIN/LOSS

TRAIL TYPE (CIRCLE ONE): ◯ **OUT & BACK** ◯ **LOOP** ◯ **ONE WAY / SHUTTLE**

📍 **THE HIKE** ☆ ☆ ☆ ☆ ☆

CITY/STATE

TRAIL(S)

START LATITUDE/LONGITUDE

TERRAIN

CEL PHONE RECEPTION/CARRIER

◯ **FIRST VISIT**   ◯ **RETURN VISIT**

PERSONAL RATING: ◯ **EASY** ◯ **INTERMEDIATE** ◯ **DIFICULT**

 COMPANION(S)

FACILITIES / WATER AVAIABILITY

TRAIL & WEATHER CONDITIONS

OBSERVANCES (WILDLIFE, NATURE, VIEWS, ETC)

NOTES FOR NEXT TIME (SHUTTLES, ENTRANCE FEES, PARKING, ROUTES, PETS, ETC.)

HIKING NOTES

TRAIL DRAWING / FAVORITE PHOTO

DATE   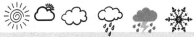 **HOT** **COLD** **MILD**

START TIME   **END TIME**

TOTAL DURATION   **TOTAL DISTANCE**

ELEVATION GAIN/LOSS

TRAIL TYPE (CIRCLE ONE):   ○ **OUT & BACK**   ○ **LOOP**   ○ **ONE WAY / SHUTTLE**

 THE HIKE ☆ ☆ ☆ ☆ ☆

CITY/STATE

TRAIL(S)

START LATITUDE/LONGITUDE

TERRAIN

CEL PHONE RECEPTION/CARRIER

○ **FIRST VISIT**   ○ **RETURN VISIT**

PERSONAL RATING: ○ **EASY**   ○ **INTERMEDIATE**   ○ **DIFICULT**

 COMPANION(S)

_____

FACILITIES / WATER AVAIABILITY

_____

TRAIL & WEATHER CONDITIONS

_____

OBSERVANCES (WILDLIFE, NATURE, VIEWS, ETC)

_____

NOTES FOR NEXT TIME (SHUTTLES, ENTRANCE FEES, PARKING, ROUTES, PETS, ETC.)

_____

HIKING NOTES

_____
_____
_____
_____
_____
_____
_____
_____
_____
_____
_____
_____

TRAIL DRAWING / FAVORITE PHOTO

Date 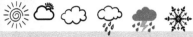 HOT COLD MILD

START TIME **END TIME**

TOTAL DURATION **TOTAL DISTANCE**

ELEVATION GAIN/LOSS

TRAIL TYPE (CIRCLE ONE): ◯ **OUT & BACK** ◯ **LOOP** ◯ **ONE WAY / SHUTTLE**

 THE HIKE ★ ★ ★ ★ ★

CITY/STATE

TRAIL(S)

START LATITUDE/LONGITUDE

TERRAIN

CEL PHONE RECEPTION/CARRIER

◯ **FIRST VISIT** ◯ **RETURN VISIT**

PERSONAL RATING: ◯ **EASY** ◯ **INTERMEDIATE** ◯ **DIFICULT**

 COMPANION(S)

FACILITIES / WATER AVAIABILITY

TRAIL & WEATHER CONDITIONS

OBSERVANCES (WILDLIFE, NATURE, VIEWS, ETC)

NOTES FOR NEXT TIME (SHUTTLES, ENTRANCE FEES, PARKING, ROUTES, PETS, ETC.)

HIKING NOTES

TRAIL DRAWING / FAVORITE PHOTO

DATE _____ 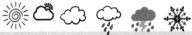 **HOT** **COLD** **MILD**

START TIME _____   **END TIME** _____

TOTAL DURATION _____   **TOTAL DISTANCE** _____

ELEVATION GAIN/LOSS _____

TRAIL TYPE (CIRCLE ONE):   ○ **OUT & BACK**   ○ **LOOP**   ○ **ONE WAY / SHUTTLE**

THE HIKE   ★ ★ ★ ★ ★

CITY/STATE _____

TRAIL(S) _____

START LATITUDE/LONGITUDE _____

TERRAIN _____

CEL PHONE RECEPTION/CARRIER _____

○ **FIRST VISIT**   ○ **RETURN VISIT**

PERSONAL RATING: ○ **EASY**   ○ **INTERMEDIATE**   ○ **DIFICULT**

 COMPANION(S) _____

_____

FACILITIES / WATER AVAIABILITY _____

_____

TRAIL & WEATHER CONDITIONS _____

_____

OBSERVANCES (WILDLIFE, NATURE, VIEWS, ETC) _____

_____

NOTES FOR NEXT TIME (SHUTTLES, ENTRANCE FEES, PARKING, ROUTES, PETS, ETC.) _____

_____

HIKING NOTES

_____
_____
_____
_____
_____
_____
_____
_____
_____
_____
_____
_____
_____
_____

TRAIL DRAWING / FAVORITE PHOTO

DATE _____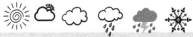

 START TIME _____ 🏁 **END TIME** _____

TOTAL DURATION _____ **TOTAL DISTANCE** _____

ELEVATION GAIN/LOSS _____

TRAIL TYPE (CIRCLE ONE): ◯ **OUT & BACK** ◯ **LOOP** ◯ **ONE WAY / SHUTTLE**

THE HIKE ⭐ ⭐ ⭐ ⭐ ⭐

CITY/STATE _____

TRAIL(S) _____

START LATITUDE/LONGITUDE _____

TERRAIN _____

CEL PHONE RECEPTION/CARRIER _____

◯ **FIRST VISIT** ◯ **RETURN VISIT**

PERSONAL RATING: ◯ **EASY** ◯ **INTERMEDIATE** ◯ **DIFICULT**

 COMPANION(S)
_____
_____

FACILITIES / WATER AVAIABILITY
_____
_____

TRAIL & WEATHER CONDITIONS
_____
_____

OBSERVANCES (WILDLIFE, NATURE, VIEWS, ETC)
_____
_____

NOTES FOR NEXT TIME (SHUTTLES, ENTRANCE FEES, PARKING, ROUTES, PETS, ETC.)
_____
_____

HIKING NOTES

TRAIL DRAWING / FAVORITE PHOTO

DATE 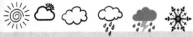 **HOT** **COLD** **MILD**

START TIME **END TIME**

TOTAL DURATION   **TOTAL DISTANCE**

ELEVATION GAIN/LOSS

TRAIL TYPE (CIRCLE ONE):   ◯ **OUT & BACK**   ◯ **LOOP**   ◯ **ONE WAY / SHUTTLE**

 ## THE HIKE   ⭐ ⭐ ⭐ ⭐ ⭐

CITY/STATE
_____

TRAIL(S)
_____

START LATITUDE/LONGITUDE
_____

TERRAIN
_____

CEL PHONE RECEPTION/CARRIER
_____

◯ **FIRST VISIT**   ◯ **RETURN VISIT**

PERSONAL RATING: ◯ **EASY**   ◯ **INTERMEDIATE**   ◯ **DIFICULT**

 COMPANION(S)
_____
_____

FACILITIES / WATER AVAIABILITY
_____
_____

TRAIL & WEATHER CONDITIONS
_____
_____

OBSERVANCES (WILDLIFE, NATURE, VIEWS, ETC)
_____
_____

NOTES FOR NEXT TIME (SHUTTLES, ENTRANCE FEES, PARKING, ROUTES, PETS, ETC.)
_____
_____

HIKING NOTES

_____
_____
_____
_____
_____
_____
_____
_____
_____
_____
_____
_____
_____
_____

TRAIL DRAWING / FAVORITE PHOTO

DATE   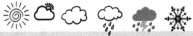 HOT COLD MILD

START TIME **END TIME**

TOTAL DURATION   **TOTAL DISTANCE**

ELEVATION GAIN/LOSS

TRAIL TYPE (CIRCLE ONE):   ◯ **OUT & BACK**   ◯ **LOOP**   ◯ **ONE WAY / SHUTTLE**

 ## THE HIKE ☆ ☆ ☆ ☆ ☆

CITY/STATE

TRAIL(S)

START LATITUDE/LONGITUDE

TERRAIN

CEL PHONE RECEPTION/CARRIER

◯ **FIRST VISIT**   ◯ **RETURN VISIT**

PERSONAL RATING: ◯ **EASY**   ◯ **INTERMEDIATE**   ◯ **DIFICULT**

 COMPANION(S)

FACILITIES / WATER AVAIABILITY

TRAIL & WEATHER CONDITIONS

OBSERVANCES (WILDLIFE, NATURE, VIEWS, ETC)

NOTES FOR NEXT TIME (SHUTTLES, ENTRANCE FEES, PARKING, ROUTES, PETS, ETC.)

HIKING NOTES

TRAIL DRAWING / FAVORITE PHOTO

DATE

START TIME   **END TIME**

TOTAL DURATION   **TOTAL DISTANCE**

ELEVATION GAIN/LOSS

TRAIL TYPE (CIRCLE ONE):   OUT & BACK   LOOP   ONE WAY / SHUTTLE

THE HIKE   ★ ★ ★ ★ ★

CITY/STATE

TRAIL(S)

START LATITUDE/LONGITUDE

TERRAIN

CEL PHONE RECEPTION/CARRIER

FIRST VISIT   RETURN VISIT

PERSONAL RATING: EASY   INTERMEDIATE   DIFICULT

 COMPANION(S)

FACILITIES / WATER AVAIABILITY

TRAIL & WEATHER CONDITIONS

OBSERVANCES (WILDLIFE, NATURE, VIEWS, ETC)

NOTES FOR NEXT TIME (SHUTTLES, ENTRANCE FEES, PARKING, ROUTES, PETS, ETC.)

HIKING NOTES

_____
_____
_____
_____
_____
_____
_____
_____
_____
_____
_____
_____

TRAIL DRAWING / FAVORITE PHOTO

DATE 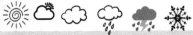 **HOT** **COLD** **MILD**

START TIME **END TIME**

TOTAL DURATION   **TOTAL DISTANCE**

ELEVATION GAIN/LOSS

TRAIL TYPE (CIRCLE ONE):   ◯ **OUT & BACK**   ◯ **LOOP**   ◯ **ONE WAY / SHUTTLE**

📍 THE HIKE   ⭐⭐⭐⭐⭐

CITY/STATE

TRAIL(S)

START LATITUDE/LONGITUDE

TERRAIN

CEL PHONE RECEPTION/CARRIER

◯ **FIRST VISIT**   ◯ **RETURN VISIT**

PERSONAL RATING: ◯ **EASY**   ◯ **INTERMEDIATE**   ◯ **DIFICULT**

 COMPANION(S)

FACILITIES / WATER AVAIABILITY

TRAIL & WEATHER CONDITIONS

OBSERVANCES (WILDLIFE, NATURE, VIEWS, ETC)

NOTES FOR NEXT TIME (SHUTTLES, ENTRANCE FEES, PARKING, ROUTES, PETS, ETC.)

HIKING NOTES

_____

_____

_____

_____

_____

_____

_____

_____

_____

_____

_____

_____

TRAIL DRAWING / FAVORITE PHOTO

DATE 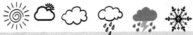 HOT COLD MILD

START TIME   **END TIME**

TOTAL DURATION   **TOTAL DISTANCE**

ELEVATION GAIN/LOSS

TRAIL TYPE (CIRCLE ONE):   OUT & BACK   LOOP   ONE WAY / SHUTTLE

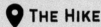 THE HIKE ⭐⭐⭐⭐⭐

CITY/STATE

TRAIL(S)

START LATITUDE/LONGITUDE

TERRAIN

CEL PHONE RECEPTION/CARRIER

    FIRST VISIT   RETURN VISIT

PERSONAL RATING: EASY   INTERMEDIATE   DIFICULT

 COMPANION(S)

FACILITIES / WATER AVAIABILITY

TRAIL & WEATHER CONDITIONS

OBSERVANCES (WILDLIFE, NATURE, VIEWS, ETC)

NOTES FOR NEXT TIME (SHUTTLES, ENTRANCE FEES, PARKING, ROUTES, PETS, ETC.)

HIKING NOTES

TRAIL DRAWING / FAVORITE PHOTO

DATE 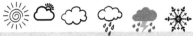 HOT COLD MILD

 START TIME   **END TIME**

TOTAL DURATION   **TOTAL DISTANCE**

ELEVATION GAIN/LOSS

TRAIL TYPE (CIRCLE ONE):   OUT & BACK   LOOP   ONE WAY / SHUTTLE

THE HIKE ⭐⭐⭐⭐⭐

CITY/STATE

TRAIL(S)

START LATITUDE/LONGITUDE

TERRAIN

CEL PHONE RECEPTION/CARRIER

   FIRST VISIT   RETURN VISIT

PERSONAL RATING: EASY   INTERMEDIATE   DIFICULT

 COMPANION(S)

FACILITIES / WATER AVAIABILITY

TRAIL & WEATHER CONDITIONS

OBSERVANCES (WILDLIFE, NATURE, VIEWS, ETC)

NOTES FOR NEXT TIME (SHUTTLES, ENTRANCE FEES, PARKING, ROUTES, PETS, ETC.)

HIKING NOTES

_____
_____
_____
_____
_____
_____
_____
_____
_____
_____
_____
_____

TRAIL DRAWING / FAVORITE PHOTO

Thank You!

We hope you enjoyed our Planner.

.

As a small familly company, your feedback is verry important to us.

Please let us know how you like our book at:

adildaisy@gmail.com

"THE EARTH HAS MUSIC FOR THOSE WHO LISTEN."

WILLIAM SHAKESPEARE

CPSIA information can be obtained
at www.ICGtesting.com
Printed in the USA
LVHW010500220221
679515LV00005B/893

9 781044 132384